B
Natural Energy

40 Simple Exercises and
Recipes for Everyday

Sandy Taikyu Kuhn Shimu

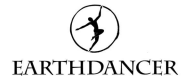

EARTHDANCER

AN INNER TRADITIONS IMPRINT

First edition 2019

Sandy Taikyu Kuhn Shimu
Boost your Natural Energy
40 Simple Exercises and Recipes for Everyday

This English edition © 2019 Earthdancer GmbH
English translation © 2019 JMS books LLP
Editing by JMS books LLP (www.jmseditorial.com)
Originally published as: *Was die Energie zum Fließen bringt:*
  Der kleine Energieratgeber für jeden Tag
World © 2013 Schirner Verlag, Darmstadt, Germany

Cover design: DesignIsIdentity.com
Cover images: Serhii Yurkiv (mountain woman),
  vectortatu (sun rays), both shutterstock.com
Typesetting and layout: DesignIsIdentity.com
Typeset in Whitman and Myriad
Printed and bound in China by Midas Printing Ltd.

ISBN 978-1-62055-974-1 (print)
ISBN 978-1-62055-975-8 (ebook)

Published by Earthdancer, an imprint of Inner Traditions
www.earthdancerbooks.com, www.innertraditions.com

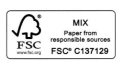

The flow
of your own heart

Open yourself to the source of your power.
Realize that everything is already present within you.

*There is nothing in excess there,
and nothing missing.*
Nothing has been achieved and nothing neglected.
There is neither right nor wrong, neither good nor bad.

If you truly follow the inner voice
*of your heart,
you will never disappoint yourself.*

Sandy Taikyu Kuhn Shimu

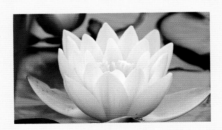

Contents

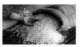

Introduction

The Chinese call it *qi*, the Japanese *ki*, and the Indians *prana*. To Christians it is "the breath of life," to Tibetans "lung," and the Greeks knew it as *pneuma*. These are all different terms for the same concept: the life energy that each individual possesses. This potential energy is shaped by your everyday routines, your lifestyle, your approach to life. Everything you think, feel, eat, and drink, not to mention the way you act, live, breathe, and speak, will affect your energy. When your energy is flowing, you feel healthy, capable, focused, happy, and balanced; your body and mind form an inseparable whole and you have access to all your power.

When your energy is blocked, you feel pain and tension. You are unhappy, irritable, nervous, unsettled, or angry, and you feel vulnerable, misunderstood, or sick. Your body and mind are no longer a whole, and everything you do costs you additional energy. Every task feels like a burden that is both exhausting and challenging.

Our energy flow will always be blocked if we direct our energy against something, when we are at odds with a set of circumstances, a situation, environment, or person; when we dig our heels in; in short, when our actions are not in harmony with what we think and feel.

Instead, become one with what you are doing, mentally and physically; accept even difficult situations, have the ability to let go, and deal with problems constructively. You will then be able to make the right decisions in accordance with your true nature. You will be living in your natural flow and everything will feel familiar and right. Of course, even this will sometimes feel like hard work; what you do will be in harmony with what you think and feel, but to achieve this, you will have to devote all your attention and commitment to finding your way back to the present and giving your mind and body a chance to reunite. You can only achieve this when you stop fighting for or against something, and let go.

Every individual can restore their flow of life energy through specific physical exercises, simple breathing techniques and meditations, and even tasty energy drinks. This little guide is a true treasure chest that will show you easy yet effective ways of exploiting your potential. All my recommendations are intended to provide support for your physical and mental well-being. They are tried and tested and have been sourced from my many years of experience and practice both as a teacher of martial arts, qigong, meditation, and yoga and as a psycholog-ical coach. However, each person will react according to their own individual energy patterns and personal capacities, so your own progress may vary and your experience will be as individ-ual as you are. This book does not claim to be a panacea and is no substitute for seeing a doctor, an alternative practitioner, or a therapist, as may be appropriate. Neither the author nor the publisher can accept any liability for damage to persons, goods, or assets.

There are a number of different ways you can work with this guide. You might decide to read it from start to finish or to search instead for exercises, techniques, or recipes that answer your immediate needs. There is a short introduction to each piece of advice and/or some background information about the topic. For some of the exercises, I have provided instructions about the number of repetitions or the duration of the routine. Please take these as guidelines rather than rules set in stone; experiment and keep an eye on how you are doing. As long as you are feeling mentally and physically well, you are on the right path. Please be aware, however, that as you begin your routine, you may experience a few minor side effects such as tiredness, as energy blocks and energy patterns dissolve and loosen. These are entirely normal reactions, and with care they can be kept to a minimum. Always do the exercises carefully and with full awareness. Leave yourself time and take baby steps, particularly if you have little or no previous experience with energy work. You can combine any of the exercises and even create your own exercise routines. I have put together a list of useful, tried-and-tested exercise routines arranged under various headings at the end of the book, and these should help to inspire you.

Remember:
Joy is the greatest source of energy!

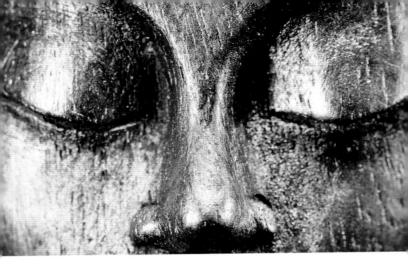

Eye bath

The eyes are considered the mirror of the soul and a picture is worth a thousand words, as the old saying goes. We often send out entirely unconscious signals with our eyes; we can look dismissive, inquisitive, reproachful, or intrigued, and our eyes can gleam, twinkle, or shine with joy, love, or happiness. We can also look sad, furious, frightened, or secretive, of course; our eyes are our window on the outside world just as much as they are the link to our inner world.

EFFECT

An eye bath will cleanse the cornea and conjunctiva and generally moisten the eye; it can be especially helpful for tired or dry eyes, or if you are suffering from an allergic reaction. An eye bath soothes mild irritations and calms and refreshes the eyes. People who spend a lot of time in front of computer screens, work in air-conditioned offices, or wear contact lenses will derive far greater benefit from an eye bath than from using conventional eye drops, as it is more effective and provides the eyes with holistic and long-lasting care.

METHOD

The first thing you will need is the eye bath itself, and this is available from most pharmacies. You can either make the solution to fill the eye bath yourself, or you can buy it at a pharmacy or any other specialist shop. Traditionally, an eye bath will call for a saline solution: dissolve a pinch of fine-grain salt in 3.5 fl oz (100 ml) lukewarm water. As this solution has the same concentration of sodium chloride as tears, it will not cause a burning sensation to the eyes. Remove your make-up, wash your hands thoroughly and take out your contact lenses. Fill the eye bath with the salt solution. Position the eye bath over one eye so that no water can leak out and tip your head back. Open your eye and slowly move your eyeball around for 30 to 60 seconds. Empty the eye bath, refill it with fresh salt solution, and repeat the procedure for the other eye. Eye lotions are available from drugstores.

My eye exercises (see p. 31) are a wonderful complement to an eye bath.

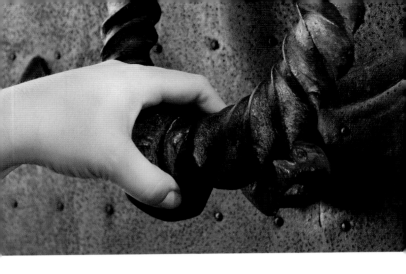

Tapping your thymus gland

BACK-GROUND The Latin word *thymus* is derived from the Greek *thymos*, meaning "life force." The thymus gland is the most important organ in the human immune system as it secretes defence hormones. It not only influences our ability to deal with burdens and assaults on our physical and emotional state but also helps us to defend ourselves successfully against attack. The thymus is located in the center of the torso behind the sternum, about 2½ inches (7 cm) beneath the throat.

EFFECT

This simple exercise relieves stress and anxiety while also boosting the body's defences. It will give you courage and drive and boost your vitality.

Children and young adults also benefit from this exercise. Activate your thymus before an exam, a job interview, or a lecture for greater composure, peace of mind, and self-assurance.

METHOD

Sit or stand upright. Use your fingertips or fists to tap on the thymus and/or sternum for 60 seconds. As you are doing this, remember to breathe regularly and tap rhythmically, adapting the intensity of the tapping to your needs and well-being. You can do this exercise several times a day. Children love to roar like Tarzan when they are activating their thymus glands!

I recommend you try body tapping (see p. 25) as a complement to this exercise.

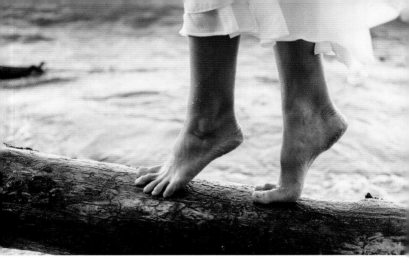

Rolling your feet

BACK-GROUND Our feet carry us through life, and a healthy person can take around 10,000 steps in a day. This is reason enough to take good care of our feet and to ensure they get enough attention and respite. There are so-called reflex zones on our feet; these are areas across the whole foot that are connected with our organs or other parts of the body via nerves, blood vessels, the lymphatic system, and the energy highways (meridians). There is a reciprocal relationship between each organ and reflex zone; each is dependent on and can influence the other.

EFFECT Rolling your feet not only improves the circulation in your limbs but also boosts blood flow in the organ or body part that is linked to the reflex zone. It is vitally important to have good circulation, as the blood carries all our body's nutrients, catabolic waste, oxygen, hormones, and antibodies (the body's defence mechanism). Regular foot massage will reduce deposits and crystallization of uric acid and other waste products, activate the body's powers of self-healing, promote bodily awareness, and ease tensions and blockages. You will also be strengthening the muscles in your feet and keeping your feet moving.

METHOD Lay a wooden roller or a plastic pipe on a flat floor; the roller should be about 1–2 inches (2.5–5 cm) in diameter and about 6–12 inches (15–30 cm) in length. You might want to place a non-slip surface underneath, such as a rubber mat or a piece of carpet. Take off your socks and begin the exercise with your left foot, rolling it across the roller for 5 minutes. Now massage your right foot, always taking care to treat the full length of your sole. You should also vigorously roll your heels, your arches, and the balls of your feet. Tip and turn your feet to reach the inside and outside edges as well. It is not unusual for the occasional spot or area to be a little (or even quite) painful at the beginning. Don't massage any harder than you can take while still feeling relaxed and with a smile on your lips. The more regularly you roll your feet, the quicker the pain will subside; when you start out, it is advisable to massage your feet every day.

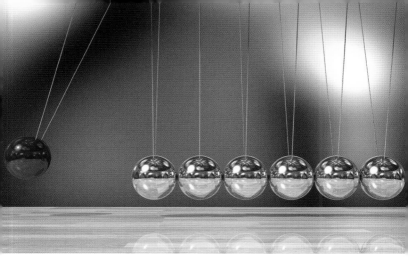

Swinging your arms

BACK-GROUND The Indian monk Bodhidharma, the founder of Chan and Zen Buddhism, is depicted in contemporary illustrations as the originator of this simple but very effective exercise taken from qigong. This practice has always been very popular in China and Taiwan, especially with older people, who gather in the park and even enjoy a chat and a laugh together as they swing their arms in unison. There are many advantages to this exercise: you don't need much space to do it, it is highly effective, and it can be carried out without prior expertise or equipment.

EFFECT

This simple exercise improves energy flow throughout the entire body, naturally reinforcing and loosening the spine, shoulders, arms, and legs, as well as your back muscles. The body relaxes, blockages are removed, and your qi can flow without let or hindrance. Swinging your arms also has a beneficial effect on your respiratory organs and your cardiovascular system.

METHOD

Stand upright, with your feet about hip- or shoulder-width apart and parallel to one another. Bend your knees slightly, with your knee joints relaxed. Alternatively, you might like to sit on an upright chair if you find standing difficult. Breathe in and out naturally through your nose throughout the entire exercise. Begin by swinging both arms forward and up until they are level with your shoulders at the front before letting them fall back past your hips. With your palms facing down, raise and release your arms like a pendulum that swings backward and forward; this will relax your mind. Continue the exercise for at least 5 minutes, concentrating on maintaining a regular, flowing rhythm, then slowly reduce the tempo until your arms are finally at rest by your sides. Enjoy the feeling for a little while.

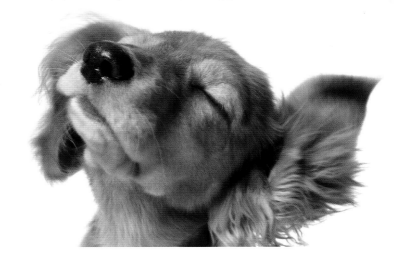

Shaking exercise

BACK-GROUND

This exercise taken from qigong is well-known and very popular in China, and has now caught on in the West as well. It is easy to do and extremely effective. In China, people often say "just shake off illnesses and worries!" and this shaking exercise is an attempt to restore the body's energy to its natural flow, casting off stale qi and taking in new qi.

EFFECT

This simple exercise reduces physical and mental tension by purifying, harmonizing, and strengthening, while also creating a path for energy through the body and dispelling fatigue. This shaking exercise is stimulating and revitalizing, and can also bring healing, vigor, and balance.

METHOD Stand upright with your feet about hip- or shoulder-width apart and parallel to one another. Bend your knees slightly, with your knee joints relaxed. Make sure you are standing in a stable position, remaining centered and well-grounded throughout the entire exercise. Close your eyes, breathing in and out naturally through the nose. Relax your shoulders and keep your arms and hands loose. Hold this position for about a minute and then begin to shake your whole body from your legs up. This shaking movement should be completely intuitive, but try to get your whole body involved; shake every part of your body, every muscle, organ, and cell. Just let go, shaking everything off, with no control, no thought, and no attempt at influencing your movements. Shake your body for at least 5 to 10 minutes before slowing your movement and then bringing your shaking to a gradual halt. Stand completely still for a few minutes, calmly enjoying the feeling. Perform this exercise once a day.

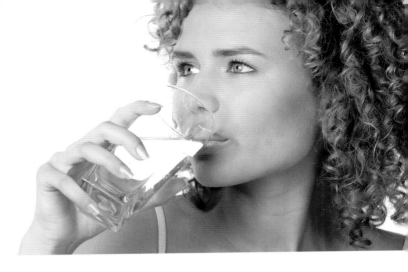

Drinking hot water

Water is the elixir of life. Drinking hot water regularly is extremely healthy and can boost your well-being considerably with its refreshing and revitalizing properties. Dehydration will soon make itself known through tiredness, loss of concentration, and irritability. As about 75 percent of the body actually consists of water, it is easy to absorb, process, and excrete. Regular consumption of hot water will lighten the load on your kidneys and liver while also topping up your body's reserves of liquids.

EFFECT Drinking hot water at intervals during the day will activate your metabolism, encourage the purification of your body, boost your digestive organs, and encourage absorption of nutrients. It warms our innards, draws out toxins, reduces weight, encourages us to pass water, and promotes the vitality and elasticity of the skin. Normal feelings of thirst and hunger will set in after a certain amount of time. In China it is thought that (excessive) hunger can often be a misunderstood indication of thirst.

METHOD Boil 4¼ pints (2 litres) of water and let it simmer at a rolling boil for about 10 minutes. Transfer the water to an insulated flask and drink about a cupful (200 ml) at a time, spread over the day. Begin in the morning, drinking one or two cupfuls (200–500 ml) on an empty stomach.

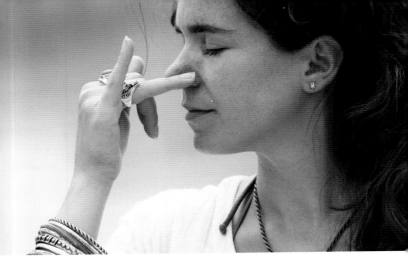

Alternate breathing

BACK-GROUND

Breath has been considered the bridge between body and mind since ancient times. We all have our own individual breathing rhythm and we normally breathe entirely unconsciously, which is why we have little control over our bodies, our minds, or our energy systems. When we relearn to breathe consciously, we gain the power to influence not only our breathing but also our minds and our energy levels.

EFFECT

This breathing exercise cleanses your system of energy channels, clearing blockages, promoting concentration, bringing balance, and restoring harmony. Alternate breathing prevents colds, allergies, asthma, and hay fever, boosts lung capacity, and provides a workout for your heart and circulation. It calms the nerves and shores up your inner peace, thereby promoting mental and physical balance.

METHOD Sit upright on a chair or on a cushion on the floor. Never try this exercise on a full stomach or if you are under time pressure. First, blow your nose (always keep a tissue handy, just in case). When carrying out the exercise, use the thumb of your right hand to close your right nostril, and the ring finger and little finger of the same hand to close your left one. Your middle finger and index finger should be bent inward to touch your palm, the correct finger position for alternate breathing. Open your nostrils and breathe in and out consciously through both nostrils. Now breathe in and close your right nostril with your thumb. Breathe out through your left nostril then inhale through the same nostril without pausing. Close your left nostril (both nostrils are now closed). Hold your breath, but avoid becoming uncomfortably short of breath. Release your thumb and breathe out through your right nostril again. Breathe in again through the same nostril without pausing, and then close it. Hold your breath again, without feeling like you are suffocating. Release your ring finger and little finger and breathe out through your left nostril. You have now done one round of alternate breathing. Do at least eight rounds, and then sit back for a couple of minutes to enjoy the feeling.

The exercises "Long-life breathing" (p. 64) and "Bumble bee breath" (p. 68) complement this exercise very well.

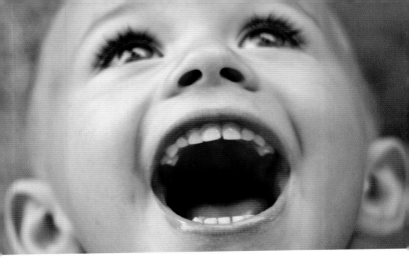

Primal scream

Letting off steam properly is very important for preserving your harmonic balance; people all too often internalize their cares and worries and "swallow" their rage and anger. They are then not only directing their energy against themselves, but introducing tension and blockages to their bodies and minds. By contrast, screaming indicates an ability to let go and to trust. If you trust yourself enough to roar really loudly, you will free yourself from pent-up feelings and sensations and also gain in self-confidence, clarity, and energy.

EFFECT

Letting out a healthy scream from the pit of your stomach releases tension, liberates blocked energies and stifled emotion, and frees you from physical pain. A primal scream of this kind will reduce stress and muscle tension, and can also help to reduce anxiety and help you let go on a mental and physical level.

METHOD

Find a place where you can scream freely in private, such as in a deserted patch of forest, in the mountains, near a waterfall, by the sea, or in the car. You can also scream into the wind. Bring your pain, frustration, or rage to mind, breathe in deeply, and let go at the top of your lungs, summoning everything that is weighing you down, depressing you, or hemming you in. Repeat the exercise until you feel freer, fresher, clearer, better, and more relaxed.

I recommend "Deep relaxation: Shavasana" (p. 74) as a complement to this exercise.

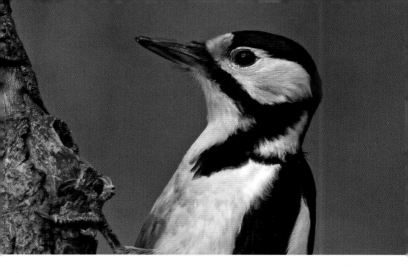

Body tapping

BACK-GROUND The Chinese term "qigong" describes working with qi, and this involves both mobile and static energy exercises. Body tapping is one of the simplest qigong exercises; it is an effective way to maintain your health and requires very little time or space (and no equipment!). Cultivating your own energy is essential; it is the only way to spot and release energy blocks in good time. In China and Taiwan, the exercise to create physical and mental harmony is also known as tapping massage. Instead of using the flat of their hands, experts will tie up a small bundle of bamboo and tap with that to enhance the effects on the body. A small bag filled with sand can also be used for tapping massage.

EFFECT

This exercise promotes blood circulation and improves the flow of qi. It revitalizes and activates the whole body and also maintains your health. After tapping your body you will feel at ease, relaxed, and refreshed; your positive strength will be activated.

METHOD

Stand upright, with your feet about hip- or shoulder-width apart and parallel to one another. Bend your knees slightly, with your knee joints relaxed. Alternatively, you can sit on a chair if you find standing difficult. Breathe in and out naturally through your nose throughout the entire exercise. Slightly cup your hand and tap all over your body, beginning with your shoulders and arms before continuing on to your chest, stomach, hips, and back. Tap on your buttocks and legs; you can of course swap the hand you are tapping with, as necessary. Instead of tapping, you can also firmly rub sensitive spots like your joints or your stomach with the flat of your hand. Take a little while to enjoy the sensation afterward.

I recommend the exercises "Washing your face" (p. 27) and "Tapping your thymus gland" (p. 11), before or after tapping, as a beneficial complement to this exercise.

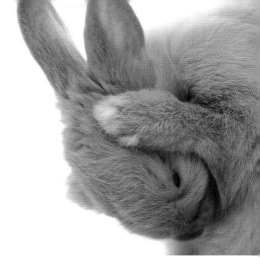

Washing your face

BACK-GROUND

This is another very easy but highly effective qigong exercise that restores the natural harmony of body and mind. When you "wash" it, your face stocks up on fresh energy, and blockages and signs of tiredness are sluiced away.

EFFECT

This exercise revitalizes and rejuvenates the face, strengthening the flow of qi and boosting your well-being. It will wake you up, encouraging clear and concentrated thought and relaxing your mind.

METHOD Sit or stand upright, and if you wear glasses, take them off. Breathe in and out naturally through your nose throughout the entire exercise. Rub your palms together until they feel pleasantly warm. Now imagine that your hands are a washcloth and "wash" or rub your whole face vigorously with your warm palms. You can also include your neck and throat if you like. You can repeat this exercise as many times a day as you like.

The two short exercises "Ear massage" (p. 54) and "Combing your hair" (p. 62) will noticeably boost your well-being.

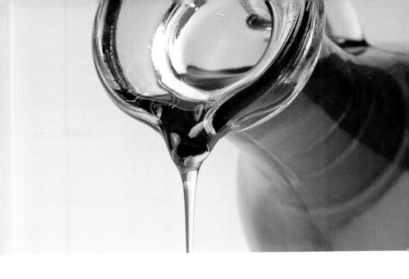

Oil pulling

BACK-GROUND

Oil pulling, also known as "kavala," was rediscovered by Russian popular medicine in the 20th century; the roots of this simple, cheap, and effective treatment lie in India and Tibet.

EFFECT

A properly conducted oil cure treatment, in which oil is pulled once a day for 4 weeks, will free the body of toxins and waste products. Oil pulling channels toxins out of the body, activates the lymphatic system, and boosts immune responses. It can help with skin conditions, headaches or toothache, muscle or joint pain, bowel, liver, and kidney complaints, and general digestive disorders.

29

METHOD As soon as you get up and before eating, place 1 tbsp of unadulterated, cold-pressed sunflower oil in your mouth. Other traditions employ olive oil or sesame oil. "Chew" the oil and strain it through your teeth without swallowing it. Keep chewing and straining until its consistency and color change; the oil is initially light yellow and free-flowing, but after use it will be milky-white and thicker in consistency. This will normally take 10 to 20 minutes. You can then spit it out into the toilet. Make sure that you do not swallow any oil, as the toxins should leave your body. Now rinse your mouth with warm water, cleanse your tongue, and clean your teeth.

I recommend the exercise "Cleansing your tongue" (p. 90) to go with this treatment.

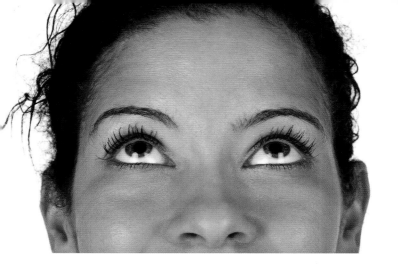

Eye exercises

Muscles like to be used and should be kept moving; being employed for their natural purpose keeps them healthy. It takes seven muscles to move each human eye. As 90 percent of our sensory stimuli are perceived through the eyes, this is reason enough to let your eyes rest and recover every now and then. Long hours spent working in front of a screen are especially bad for our eyes and can result in tension, sore or dry eyes, or a decline in visual acuity, not to mention headaches or stiff necks. Staring at a smartphone for hours on end or watching too much TV is also bad for the eyes over the long term, and this is why it is important both to give your eye muscles a regular workout and to allow them to relax.

EFFECT

These exercises are a workout for your eye muscles and will maintain and improve your vision. They are also useful for tired or dry eyes and will get your qi flowing again.

METHOD

1. Rub your palms together until they are pleasantly warm. Place your palms very gently over your closed eyes for about 30 seconds; your eyes will enjoy the warmth and the darkness.

2. Have a couple of good yawns; this is a natural way of moistening your eyes. Alternatively (or additionally!), you can repeatedly blink very fast.

3. Keeping your head still, look as far as possible to the left eight times, and then as far as possible to the right eight times. Now look up eight times, and down eight times. Roll your eyes in each direction eight times. Finish by describing a lemniscate eight times with your eyes.

4. Let your eyes wander across the room, focusing on objects at different distances.

5. Now look out of the window. Look into the distance and then at an object just outside the window before looking back out into the distance once more.

6. Repeat steps 1 and 2.

7. To finish, keep your eyes closed for a few seconds or minutes.

I recommend an "Eye bath" (p. 9) to complement this treatment.

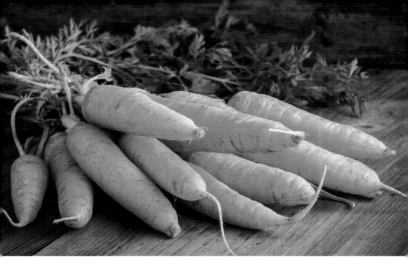

Energy drink

BACK-GROUND

This energy drink comes from Ayurveda, Indian teachings on health and healing, and tastes delicious. The juice is quick and simple to prepare, and is very easy to digest.

EFFECT

Ginger is considered the king of Ayurvedic spices. It gets the digestive juices flowing, boosts gut flora, lowers cholesterol levels and blood pressure, warms and stimulates, channels away toxins, and provides support and strength when you have a cold. Beets contain plenty of valuable vitamins, have a high iron content, and cleanse the blood and gut. Carrots are noted for their high content of vitamins, nutrients, and fiber, while cardamom is good for the digestion, neutralizes mucus, and gives you a shot of vitality, promoting clear thinking and banishing tiredness. Lemons contain lots of vitamin C, and the acid they contain revives and stimulates you, boosting your immune response and your digestion. Maple syrup is a wonderful delivery system for energy when you are feeling weak and weary.

Ingredients

- 3 carrots
- 1 beet
- ½-inch (1 cm) slice of fresh ginger root
- ½ tbsp lemon juice
- 1 pinch ground cardamom
- ½ tbsp maple syrup

METHOD

Juice the carrots, the beet, and the ginger root, then add the lemon juice, cardamom, and maple syrup. Stir everything together and enjoy this energy drink straight away.

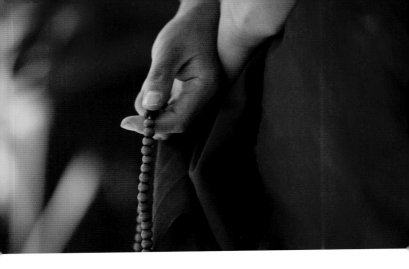

OM: A word of power

BACK-GROUND

OM (AUM) is a mantra, a word with power. It is the original sound of the cosmos, a transcendental mystical syllable. OM is the sound of the absolute and symbolizes the unity of all being.

EFFECT

Reciting or chanting the word OM promotes your inner equilibrium and ability to concentrate. It strengthens your primal energy and clarity and is an aid against depression. In addition, it will lead you to inner peace and harmony while bringing strength and energy. The mantra OM brings body and mind back into the present and unites them.

METHOD

Sit on a cushion on the floor or on a chair, or stand upright. Close your eyes and consciously breathe calmly and deeply, inhaling and exhaling a few times. Be aware of your body and your mental state without judgment. Now breathe in very deeply and chant the word OM. Try to breathe out for as long as possible, without feeing cramped up or becoming out of breath. Repeat this at least five times before returning to your natural breathing pattern, and take a moment to enjoy the feeling. You can repeat this chant (recitation) as many times as you like every day; the more you practice, the stronger the effect will be.

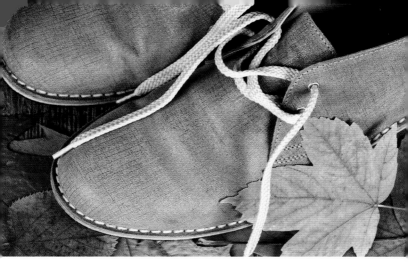

Walking backward

We normally only ever walk forward, but it sometimes does us good to change our perspective and use other muscle groups. Looking at things differently is extremely good training for the senses. There is an Asian proverb that says "100 steps backward are worth more than 1,000 steps forward," and walking backward is very popular with the Chinese and Japanese in particular, where it is practiced in groups or individually. You can walk in a straight line or a circle, and advanced students will even go upstairs backward. Other systems, such as yoga, have reverse positions known as inversions, and their positive benefits to practitioners are well known.

EFFECT

This exercise trains your coordination and concentration abilities by linking the left and right halves of the brain. It boosts every sense, stimulates your imagination, and builds up muscles that are neglected when you walk forward. Walking backward trains your hearing and will improve your balance and benefit your back, knees, and hips. It reverses the normal flow of things and has a positive and strengthening effect on the energy channels within the whole body. This exercise has a relaxing, balancing, and beneficial effect on the mind.

METHOD

Before you start practicing this exercise, make sure you are working in a safe environment. Move any dangerous objects to one side and keep away from roads or places without a clear all-round view. Begin with small, slow steps, and walk in a large circle, always resisting the temptation to turn your head and look behind you. Try to hear and feel how and where you are walking. As you practice and your confidence in your ability increases, you will be able to walk longer distances outdoors in a straight line. Always remember to breathe calmly and easily, and walk for as long as you feel good, with no tension in body or mind.

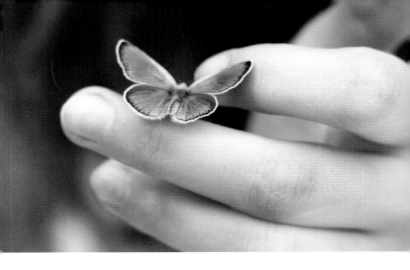

The butterfly finger game

An adult human is made up of 206 bones. Each hand has 27 bones, so a quarter of all the bones in our bodies are to be found in our two hands. Traditional Chinese medicine (TCM) makes use of this fact and has developed a special qigong system of finger exercises that provides positive support in maintaining health and helping the recuperation process of both body and mind.

This simple exercise boosts the heart and circulatory system, refreshing the mind, training the brain, and activating energy and the flow of qi in the whole body.

METHOD Place your two palms flat on your chest next to one another, with the fingertips pointing upward. Spread your fingers slightly. Move your little fingers slightly so that they overlap, swapping over so that first the right one is on top, then the left. Repeat this ten times. Repeat this movement with your ring, middle, and index fingers, and then with your thumbs. Overlap each pair of fingers ten times, breathing calmly and regularly, and relaxing the muscles in your face. You can do this finger exercise sitting, standing, or even while you walk.

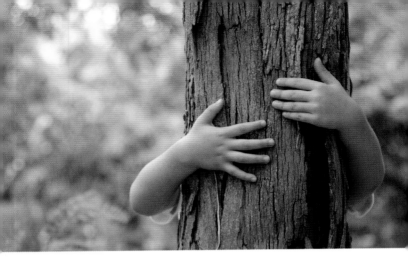

Standing like a tree

BACKGROUND

Dating back to the Yellow Emperor, who lived in China more than 4,000 years ago, this exercise is used to this day in Chinese martial arts and healing. Standing like a tree is considered a key element of energy use, and masters in a range of different disciplines generally make their students practice this posture for weeks or months before they teach them stances involving movement taken from qigong, tai chi, or wushu (kung fu).

EFFECT

Standing like a tree strengthens your bones, your body's defences, your stamina, and your ability to concentrate, as well as boosting your heart and circulation. This silent exercise relaxes and calms the mind, as it increases the oxygen supply to your cells and raises energy levels in your entire body. Your breathing rate will drop as you practice this position, and physical and mental blockages will fall away. It is said there are five regulations brought about by this exercise: regulation of body, breath, mind, consciousness (imagination), and energy.

METHOD

Stand upright on a flat floor, with your feet about hip- or shoulder-width apart. Bend your knees slightly, with your knee joints relaxed. Angle your pelvis to prevent your back from arching inward; your whole spine will now be vertical. Its normal double-S curve has been straightened to allow the qi to flow better during the exercise. Draw your chin back gently in order to straighten your cervical vertebrae. Relax your facial features and breathe through your nose. Now raise your arms in front of your chest, with your palms facing toward your torso (about level with your sternum), your fingers pointing toward one another, and your elbows angled outward. Try to keep your shoulders as relaxed as possible. Imagine you are hugging a mighty tree or holding a large ball in your arms. When you begin training, start by standing motionless for about a minute; with practice, you can increase the duration of the exercise to up to 10 minutes. When you are finished, drop your arms slowly and bring them back to your sides. Relax and enjoy the sensation for a little while.

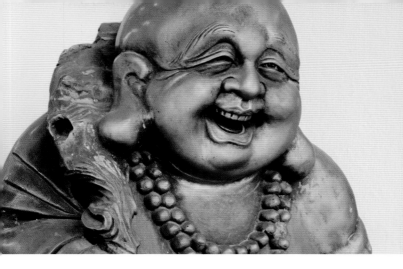

The power of a smile

There is an Indian proverb that says "the smile you send out returns to you." Old Taoist sources similarly ascribe positive responses of both body and mind to smiling. The power of a conscious smile can get the energy flowing in the body again and bring the mind consolation, calm, good cheer, and positive thoughts.

This highly effective technique allows you to boost your energy and get it flowing again. This exercise tweaks your physical and mental constitution while also helping to bring balance and harmony to your emotions and feelings, and thus to your inner equilibrium. Smile yourself happy; inner and outer calm begin with a smile.

43

METHOD

Sit upright on a chair or cushion, or on the floor. Close your eyes, breathing in and out naturally and calmly through your nose. Now begin to smile. Your brain will register the muscle activity in your face and still produce happiness hormones, irrespective of whether your smile is "natural and real" or "conscious and contrived." You will notice that something is changing within you. Now transfer this positive energy to your whole body. Try to smile for between 1 and 3 minutes. You can also get into the habit of checking yourself during the day and make a conscious effort to smile every now and again.

I recommend the exercise "Emotions in balance" (p. 60) to complement this technique.

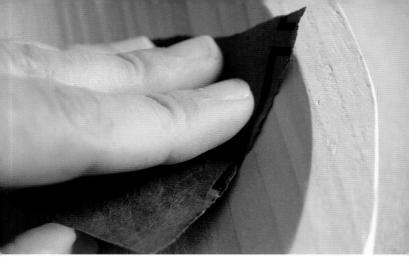

Rubbing your fingernails

BACKGROUND

We normally look after our nails by cleaning, cutting, and filing them. We push back the cuticles and treat the nails with care products such as nail oil; we make their surfaces beautiful with colored or neutral polish. We generally forget, however, to look after their energy. There is a simple method in qigong to strengthen the qi of your fingernails.

EFFECT

This exercise promotes blood flow, activates your nerves, and boosts your brain activity. It encourages nail growth, strengthens your nails, and stimulates hair growth. The energy in your fingers, hands, arms, and shoulders will also be activated, and any blockages or tension will be swept aside.

 METHOD Place your fingernails together, index fingernail to index fingernail, etc. Your hands will almost close into fists as you do this. Rub your fingernails together, all at the same time, for 3 to 5 minutes, then relax and enjoy the sensation for a little while.

To complement this technique, you might like to try out "The butterfly finger game" (p. 39).

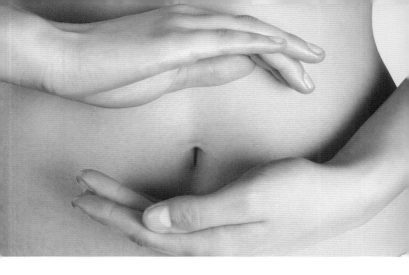

Belly massage

BACK-GROUND The belly is considered the center of the body in most Asian healing; as the seat of the body's vital spirits and the center of inner strength, it is the source of your vital energy. It is also the point where emotions, sensations, and feelings collect, and it is said that intuitive decisions are made with your "gut." There is also an important energy center in the belly, known in Chinese as "dantian," in Japanese as "hara," and in Indian culture as the "manipura chakra" or "solar plexus chakra."

EFFECT

Belly massage relaxes, warms, detoxifies, and reduces tension. It improves blood flow within the abdomen, and promotes sleep, inner calm, and contentment, as well as encouraging mental clarity and centeredness.

METHOD

You can practice this exercise sitting, standing, or lying down. Rub a few drops of olive or almond oil into your hands, making sure your palms are not cold. If they are, rub them together until they feel pleasantly warm. Now place both your hands on your belly and pause for a moment. Begin massaging by making little clockwise circles around your navel, making the circles larger and larger until you reach your ribcage and pubis. Try to use the full width of your palm. Make a total of 36 clockwise circles on the outward spiral, pressing down firmly. Then make 24 anticlockwise circles as you return to the center, this time with soft pressure, allowing your hands to travel in ever-decreasing circles. Place your hands one on top of the other, about an inch or so (2–3 cm) beneath your navel, and let them rest there for a few minutes. Repeat the exercise two or three times.

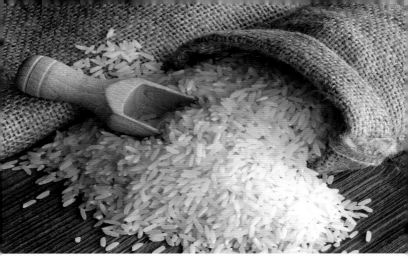

Buddha's rice soup

Soups are very popular in Asia, and in China and Taiwan people enjoy "shi fan," a watery rice porridge with little spicy or sweet morsels in it. In general, hot food strengthens your inner core and your digestion, as well as imparting physical and mental strength. The Buddha is also supposed to have said the following about rice soup:

"Rice soup brings ten gifts: life and beauty, ease and strength, it banishes hunger, thirst, and wind; it cleanses the bladder and the kidneys; and it promotes digestion."

He is also said to have praised a soup enriched with milk and honey as the healthiest food.

EFFECT This special rice soup is said to have fortifying, purifying, detoxifying, and cleansing properties. If eaten regularly, Buddha's rice soup is also thought to soothe stomach and bowel complaints, relieve allergies, and ease muscle and joint stiffness. This soup is particularly suited as a breakfast food as it will give you energy for the whole day, it won't overload your body, it is highly nutritious, and it is easily digestible. Rice soups that have been cooked for a long time also strengthen and activate the inner core and the immune system.

Ingredients

- Rice and water (1:6 ratio)
- Fresh organic milk
- Butter or ghee/clarified butter
- Honey
- Salt

METHOD The amount of water used will determine how thick the porridge/soup becomes. Don't use too much rice, as it will swell up considerably. Place the rice and water in a heavy-bottomed pan with a tight-fitting lid. After briefly bringing the rice to a boil, it is important to simmer it on the lowest possible heat for 2 to 4 hours. This will ensure it doesn't catch or burn. The longer the rice soup cooks, the more it will strengthen your qi and your blood. If you want to eat the rice soup for breakfast, you can cook it the previous evening and reheat it gently in the morning. To finish, add milk, butter or ghee, honey, and a little salt, and then add further seasoning to taste.

Vegans can replace the milk with soy or rice milk, the butter with vegetable margarine, and the honey with maple syrup or agave syrup. Fruit compote also goes very well with Buddha's rice soup in the mornings. After meals, try chewing on a teaspoon of a spice mixture consisting of, for example, aniseed, fennel, and cumin seeds; this boosts your digestion and neutralizes your mouth.

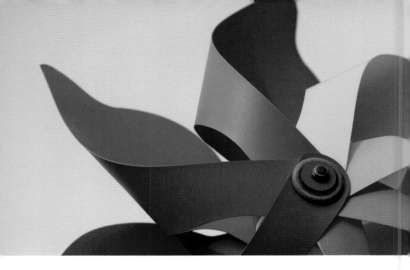

The microcosmic orbit

BACK-GROUND The microcosmic orbit is an essential Taoist exercise taken from inner alchemy and is part of silent qigong practice. Visualization is used to channel energy in the body and the two central meridians (the principal energy channels) are connected with one another. These are the *ren mai* (the servant or conception vessel), located in the center of the body at the front, and the *du mai* (the governing vessel), located in the center of the body at the back. The two forces of yin (the female dynamic) and yang (the male dynamic) are harmoniously balanced in the circulation of energy, which has a positive effect on mind and body.

EFFECT

This exercise relaxes and cleanses the body, promoting mental clarity and harmony. Energy blocks are cleared and the qi is boosted and activated.

METHOD

You can practice this exercise while sitting, standing, lying down, or walking; I recommend you start by practicing in a sitting position. Keep your spine vertical. Close your eyes and place your tongue against your upper palate. Relax your facial muscles and breathe in and out through your nose throughout the exercise. Imagine that you are sending your inner energy on a journey, an inner circulation. You can also imagine a white light or a white ball that you are propelling down the middle of your body. Begin an inch or so (2–3 cm) below the navel. Breathe in, and then move your qi across your perineum, your sacrum, and your spine, moving upward to the back of your neck and the top of your head. Breathe out and guide your energy onward, across your forehead and your third eye, and down past your upper palate and the tip of your tongue to your throat. Continue on past your sternum and navel back to the starting point, the energy center below your navel. Don't practice this circulation so fast that it leaves you out of breath; at first, you may have to take a break at some point. Do the exercise for as long as you can devote your attention and concentration to guiding your energy, but for at least nine circuits.

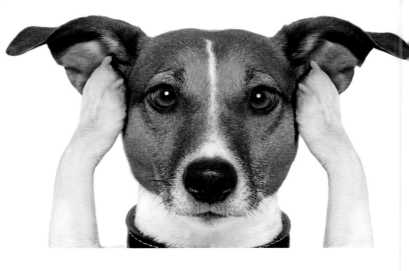

Ear massage

BACK-GROUND

TCM, or Traditional Chinese Medicine, identifies more than 100 acupuncture points in the ear, and according to the theory of reflex zone therapy, all the organs and extremities of the human body are mapped in the ear. Imagine the outer ear as a human, crouched in an upside-down, embryonic pose; the earlobe represents the head, and the edge of the ear the spine.

EFFECT

Ear massage activates your vital energy, gets the circulation up to speed, promotes concentration, stimulates the body's self-healing abilities, and has a positive effect on every organ and body part.

METHOD

Massage both ears at the same time. Starting with the earlobes, knead and rub the whole surface of your ears as firmly as possible, using thumbs, index fingers, and middle fingers. Don't forget the cartilage. To finish, fold each ear in half in the middle, pull the earlobe down, and twist your ears one way then the other. This short ear massage will only take a minute or two.

The exercise "Washing your face" (p. 27) is a wonderful complement to this technique.

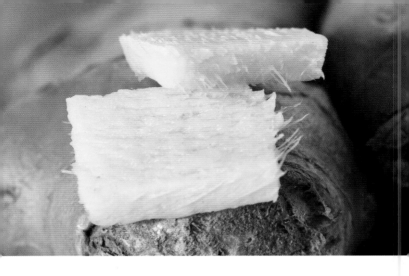

Power drink

BACK-GROUND This power drink is also taken from Ayurveda. The knowledge (*veda*) about living a long and healthy life (*ayus*) comes from India, and considers human beings to be a union of body, mind, and spirit. The power drink encourages and activates energy in the body and the mind, and all the ingredients are easily available. It is both very quick to make and extremely tasty.

EFFECT Lemons contain lots of vitamin C. This acid revitalizes, stimulates, and supports your immune system and digestion, and oranges have properties that strengthen the body and activate the digestion. Ginger stokes your digestive fires, is good for your gut flora, and reduces both your cholesterol levels and blood pressure. It has a warming and stimulating effect, sluices away toxins, and plays a supportive and strengthening role when you catch a cold or similar. Cardamom promotes digestion, neutralizes phlegm, and has an invigorating impact on your vitality. Black pepper reduces inflammation and has a soothing and supportive influence on every part of your digestive system. Brown whole cane sugar brings warmth and balance and has a gently alkalizing effect on the body.

Ingredients

- ¼ cup (60 ml) fresh lemon juice (about 1 lemon)
- ⅔ cup (150 ml) freshly squeezed sweet orange juice (about 2 oranges)
- 3 pints (1.5 l) water (or still mineral water)
- 2 tsp freshly grated ginger root
- 4 cardamom pods
- ¼–½ tsp black pepper
- 4 tbsps whole cane sugar

METHOD

Mix the water with the lemon and orange juice, then add the ginger. Pick out the cardamom seeds from the husk and grind them to a fine powder with the peppercorns using a mortar and pestle. Add the spices and the whole cane sugar to the drink, stir well, and enjoy. The mixture should ideally be consumed at room temperature.

Top tip

You can use apple juice instead of orange juice, and you might also like to try the "Energy drink" (p. 33) and the "Fitness drink" (p. 70).

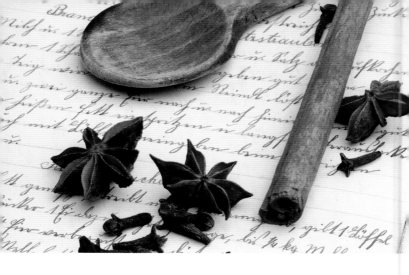

Nerve biscuits

Our diet should be healthy and delicious while also protecting and revitalizing our minds and bodies. These biscuits are very tasty and will bring your mood back on to an even keel.

EFFECT

It has been said that these biscuits have a restorative effect on your nerves; eating a few nerve biscuits will purify your senses, bring calm and balance, and restore joy to your mind. Cinnamon is warming and relaxing, stabilizes the circulation, and has a positive influence on your blood sugar levels. It helps with stomach and intestinal complaints, functions as a cleanser, and puts you in a good mood. Cloves have antibacterial properties and promote digestion. Nutmeg has an aphrodisiac effect, relieves cramps, and opens the heart, while almonds are renowned for their cholesterol-lowering properties. Spelt is easy to digest and has an alkalizing effect on the body.

Ingredients:

- 3 ⅓ cups (14 oz/400 g) spelt flour
- 1 cup (9 oz/250 g) butter, softened (vegetable margarine)
- generous ¾ cup (5 oz/ 150 g) whole cane sugar
- 1 ⅔ cups (7 oz/200 g) ground almonds
- 2 eggs, beaten
- 4 tsps (20 g) ground cinnamon
- 4 tsps (20 g) grated nutmeg
- 1 tsp (5 g) ground cloves
- 1 pinch salt

METHOD

Place the flour in a large bowl or directly on to the work surface. Cut the softened butter into small cubes and scatter over the flour. Add the whole cane sugar, the ground almonds, the eggs (vegans can use 3 tbsp apple puree), and all the spices, then mix/knead the mixture into a dough. Leave the dough to chill in the refrigerator for 30 minutes, then roll it out to a thickness of about ¼ inch (5mm) and cut it out into any shapes you like. Arrange the biscuits on a baking tray lined with baking parchment and place on the middle shelf of an oven preheated to 350°F (180°C). Bake for between 10 and 15 minutes, keeping a close eye on the biscuits the first time you bake them. Eat a maximum of four biscuits a day, depending on the size of the biscuits you have made; children should be allowed one biscuit a day.

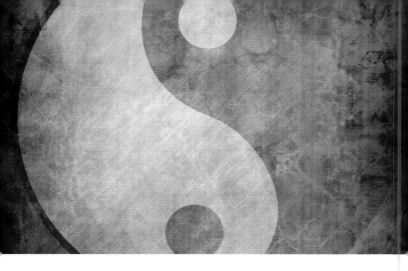

Emotions in balance

BACK-GROUND
This simple exercise is taken from the Buddhist tradition. It can be understood and practiced as a meditation or mindfulness exercise. Such techniques have also been called "exercises to unfold the heart," as they train and educate both heart and mind in equal measure. This technique in particular is about healing rifts and disagreements that have arisen with or because of other people.

EFFECT
This subtle exercise promotes insight, understanding, and wisdom, while cultivating the four great and immeasurable virtues: loving kindness, compassion, empathetic joy, and equanimity. It will

bring calm and balance to your mind and create natural and healthy harmony in your feelings, sensations, and emotions.

 METHOD Perform this exercise while seated; experienced practitioners can adopt their preferred meditation posture. Make sure the atmosphere is calm and pleasant; you might like to light a candle and burn a little incense. Switch off any potential distractions, such as your phone, and avoid background music. Allow yourself to be completely absorbed in the following mental exercise.

Imagine a person who has annoyed, disappointed, hurt, or offended you, and recite the following sentences:
- *In breathing in, I take from you everything* about you that annoys me.
- *In breathing out, I give you everything* that I would like to see in you.

Now be very precise about what annoys you and what you would like, such as:
- *When breathing in:* "I take your arrogance from you."
- *When breathing out*: "I give you the gift of grace and modesty."

Focusing on one person, repeat the sentences and do the exercise for 5 to 10 minutes or for as long as you can maintain concentration.

I recommend trying the exercise "The power of a smile" (p. 43) to complement this technique.

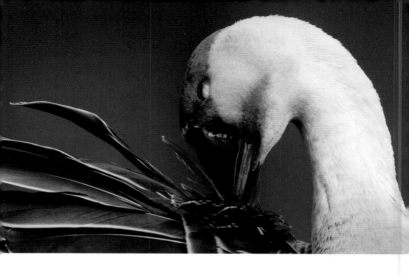

Combing your hair

Qigong is renowned for the many individual, short, and yet highly effective exercises it provides. Combing your hair is one such classic exercise. Combing addresses numerous acupuncture points on the scalp, and blockages in the head are cleared simply and effectively as the qi is allowed to flow again. In TCM the seat of the mind is located in the heart (Chinese: "shen"), that is, the heart and mind have a reciprocal relationship. This exercise thus permits us to have a direct influence on heart and mind. What is more, all yang meridians (energy channels) begin or end at the head, so all the organs of the body will be positively influenced.

EFFECT

This simple exercise activates the circulatory system and energy flow in the head, stimulating your ability to concentrate. This creates mental clarity and presence in the moment. If this technique is practiced regularly (daily, for example), hair loss and headache can be alleviated.

METHOD

You can try this exercise either standing or sitting. Using both hands simultaneously, comb your entire scalp with your fingernails, stroking from your hairline on your forehead over your whole head and down to the back of your neck. Trace consistent lines from front to back, moving a little further out with each line until you reach your ears. Make sure you use all your fingers. Repeat the combing procedure nine times, gently stroking your head with the flats of your hands for the last repetition. Now shake out your hands vigorously and repeat the procedure three times.

"Washing your face" (p. 27) and "Ear massage" (p. 54) exercises are a wonderful complement to this technique.

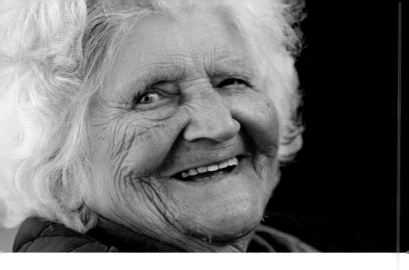

Long-life breathing

BACK-GROUND

We can survive about three weeks without solid food and around three days without liquids, but we can only survive for about three minutes without oxygen, so it will come as no surprise that breathing exercises can play an important part in maintaining physical and mental health.

EFFECT

Long-life breathing provides the entire body with oxygen. Directing your attention to these three areas of the body creates an awareness of the unique way you breathe. This breathing technique thus renders your individual breathing tangible and perceptible, trains your perceptive faculties, and has a direct effect on the nervous system. Your thoughts will be at peace, your mind can expand, and your creativity will be heightened.

METHOD Sit upright on a chair or on a cushion on the floor. Close your eyes. Breathe in and out through your nose only. Breathe a third of your respiratory capacity into your belly. Breathe the next third into your side ribs and lower back, that is, the kidney area. Breathe the last third into your chest and upper back without lifting your shoulders. Breathe out calmly from top to bottom, without tipping your torso forward or letting your chest or shoulders slump. Practice this kind of breathing for 5 to 10 minutes, making sure you don't get out of breath and remaining calm and relaxed, both mentally and physically. Enjoy the feeling for a few minutes afterward.

I recommend "Alternate breathing" (p. 21) and "Bumble bee breath" (p. 68) exercises as a complement to this technique.

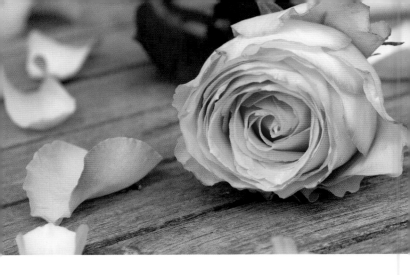

A bath for the senses

BACKGROUND Essential oils are highly effective plant extracts. When used correctly in a targeted manner, they can have a beneficial effect on our mood and our bodies. Essential oils are not only absolutely perfect for scenting rooms or as an additive for massage oils, they can also be added to your bathwater. Only buy and use 100 percent natural and purely organic oils.

EFFECT ■ *A refreshing bath with essence of lemon* will invigorate, stimulate, prepare you to tackle anything, and give your circulation a boost.

■ *A bath to treat colds with essence of spruce* is useful at the first sign of a cold. It will have a beneficial effect on muscle and limb pain, and achieves positive results with slight headaches.

■ *A get-up-and-go bath with essence of rosemary* invigorates, banishes tiredness, and gives you a shot of energy.

■ *A relaxation bath with essence of lavender* calms and harmonizes, bringing positivity and balance.

■ *A caring bath with essence of roses* will look after your skin and bring equilibrium to your psyche, helping to restore your inner balance.

■ *A relieving bath with essence of chestnut* will restore well-being and ease to the body, regenerating you and building up resources.

METHOD

Mix 5–10 drops of essential oil with 4 tbsps milk, cream, or a top-quality bath oil. This is very important, as essential oils will not combine with water without a carrier substance that contains fat! In general, you should be quite sparing with essential oils, as using too much can irritate your skin or airways. The water temperature shouldn't exceed 100°F (38°C). Don't add the mixture to the water too early and enjoy your bath for 10 to 20 minutes. Treat yourself to a little quiet time afterward and drink a refreshing cup of tea.

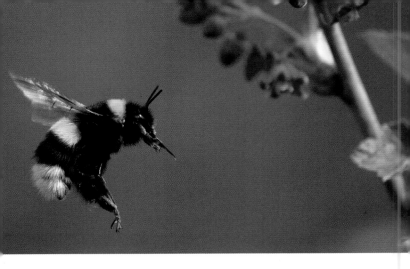

Bumble bee breath

BACK-GROUND Our breathing is influenced by a range of different external and internal factors. In general, we can use our breath to work out how things stand with our mental and physical health. Negative thoughts will make our breathing light and shallow, while positive thoughts will make it broad, open, and large. By the same token, calm, deep, flowing breathing will of course have just as great an influence on our mind as hesitant, superficial, irregular breathing. Bumble bee breath or humming like a bee is a simple and effective breathing technique.

EFFECT

This breathing technique calms the nerves and settles your thoughts. It alleviates mental tension, promotes concentration, and restores natural balance to both body and mind. This exercise will improve and strengthen your voice and increase your breathing capacity. It is good preparation for meditation and will help if you suffer from anxiety, as it fills your heart and mind with joy.

METHOD

This exercise can be done while either sitting or standing. Make sure your spine is upright. Seal your ears by raising your arms and holding your outer ears closed with thumb and index finger. Keep your elbows tucked into your sides throughout the exercise. Make sure your shoulders are relaxed. Shut your eyes and breathe in through your nose. Breathe out through your nose, making a sustained, level humming sound like a bumble bee. Do this for five to ten breaths. Release your ears, relax your arms, and enjoy the sensation for a few breaths.

"Alternate breathing" (p. 21) and "Long-life breathing" (p. 64) exercises are a wonderful complement to this technique.

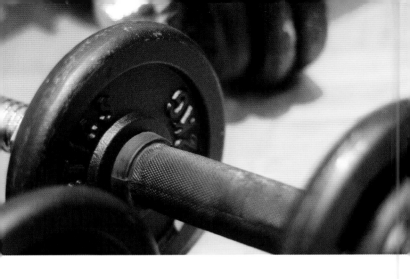

Fitness drink

BACK-GROUND
Home-made drinks whipped up with fruit or vegetables are an excellent source of vital nutrients and will supply just the kick you need at any time of the year. It is a real joy to prepare something healthy and tasty yourself, with no flavor enhancers or additives. This juice is particularly suitable for a spring detox and purification regime. It is both very tasty and quick to make.

EFFECT
Dandelion leaves are particularly rich in minerals and trace elements. They promote digestion and stimulate the metabolism. Flower pollen boosts the elasticity of the skin, strengthens nails and hair, and has a detoxifying effect. It also has a positive influence

on gut flora, shores up your immune responses, and prevents disease. Apples boost the body's performance levels and keep the mind fit and awake. Bursting with vitamins, they stimulate bowel activity, while oranges promote the metabolism of fat. They contain lots of powerful antioxidants and encourage detoxification of the body. Honey has a calming and relaxing effect, strengthening the nerves and stimulating digestion.

Ingredients

- 1 handful of young dandelion leaves
- 1 orange
- 1 apple
- ½ cup (125 ml) milk or kefir
- 1 tsp flower pollen
- Honey

METHOD Wash the dandelion leaves and cut them into strips. Juice the oranges, quarter the apples, and trim out the core. Place all the ingredients in a blender and liquidize until smooth, or use an immersion blender. Sweeten the drink with honey to taste, and enjoy this fitness drink!

Top tip

Vegans can substitute soy or rice milk for the milk or kefir and maple syrup for the honey.

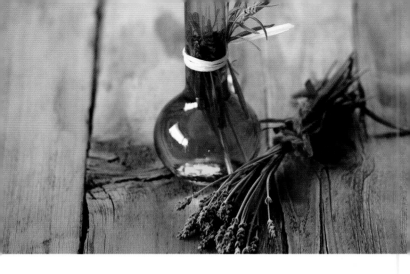

Body massage with oil

BACK-GROUND

This oil massage technique originates in Ayurvedic medicine and is considered one of the most important and fundamental therapeutic approaches for a very wide range of complaints; it is described as a key element of massage in Ayurveda and is commonly used at spas in India and Sri Lanka.

EFFECT

The results of this massage are so astonishing that you will soon be hooked. It has a holistic effect, balancing, detoxifying, and calming the nervous system. It also helps with insomnia, clears your mind, and nourishes your skin.

METHOD

You can perform this oil massage either sitting or standing. Use matured sesame oil or even olive oil. If you suffer from allergies or skin problems, use a massage oil that suits your skin type. Only buy organically grown plant-based oils. Always massage calmly, attentively, slowly, and with gentle pressure from your whole hand, not just the fingertips. The best approach is to apply slightly warmed oil evenly to the whole body, including the entire head and face, at the start of the massage. All joints should be massaged with circular movements, while muscles are treated with an upward and downward stroking motion. The massage will last for about 10 to 15 minutes, and you will need about 2¼–3½ fl oz (50–100 ml) of oil. Afterward, it is important that you leave the oil to soak in for about 15 to 25 minutes before having a shower. This will allow enough time for your body to absorb the oil and for the massage to take full effect. There is no need to use soap to wash off the oil, hot water will suffice.

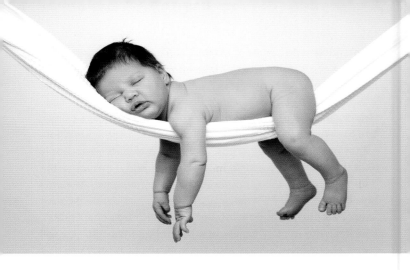

Deep relaxation: Shavasana

BACK-GROUND

"Shavasana" is a term taken from Sanskrit to describe one of the most important exercises (*asanas*) in yoga. Shavasana is a method for achieving deep relaxation in a supine position. It is considered a symbol of letting go completely and works like a fountain of youth for body and mind.

EFFECT

This simple exercise results in deep physical and mental relaxation, with a conscious letting go that imparts an attitude of silent consciousness throughout both body and mind. Physical and mental activity is calmed, allowing recent experiences to be processed and integrated. Stress hormones are reduced and happiness hormones released.

 Lie flat on your back on a level, not too soft surface. Arrange your body as neutrally and sym-
metrically as possible. Stretch out your spine and
extend your arms at an angle of about 45° from
your torso, palms facing up. Your legs should lie about hip-width apart, with your feet pointing outward in a relaxed V-position. Keep your head straight. Close your eyes and consciously relax your facial muscles, jaw, tongue, and throat. Now stop moving. Tell yourself to relax. Say in your thoughts: "My whole body is calm and relaxed. My whole body is pleasantly heavy and warm. I am relaxing my right palm. I am relaxing my left palm. I am relaxing my right sole. I am relaxing my left sole. I am relaxing my solar plexus." Let your breathing flow freely and naturally throughout the exercise. Stay still for 5 to 20 minutes. Try to remain alert, but silence your thoughts. Physically and mentally let go of everything, without falling asleep. Enjoy this moment of release, calm, and mindfulness.

Top tip
....

If you wish, place a support cushion under your knees and a small pillow under the back of your neck. An eye pillow can be very pleasant and will help you relax. If you tend to feel the cold, cover yourself with a light blanket.

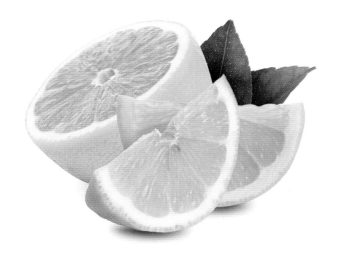

Liver cleanse

In TCM, the liver and its partner organ, the gall
bladder, are associated with the element of wood
and the season of spring in the Phases of Transfor-
mation. Wood is thus an element that also symbolizes freshness, vigor, new beginnings, tolerance, starting
journeys, motion, creativity, growth, strength, life, dynamism,
and decisiveness. The liver is responsible for the smooth flow
of energy (qi) within the entire body, although it has also been
called a "general" that takes charge of the "attacks," "defences,"
and "protection" of the body's realm. The emotions of rage and
anger are also linked to the liver.

EFFECT

This spring detox regenerates the liver, harmonizes body and mind, and activates new energy. A liver cleanse will have positive results for all the body parts you use to get about, as well as for your sight. It will also relieve the burden on your gut, purify and detoxify your system, and purge waste. Stirred-up emotions will come to rest and blockages clear. Your skin will improve and you can bid farewell to headaches, bowel conditions, and insomnia. This liver cleanse will also boost your immune defences and your decisiveness, and will activate your powers of self-healing. During this purification cure, you will experience normal detoxification symptoms such as shivering and increased tiredness; the whole process takes 7 days, but it is well worth it!

How to make your special "liver lemonade"

- 1 cup (8 fl oz/250 ml) still mineral water
- Juice of 1 lemon or lime
- Pinch of cayenne pepper
- 1–2 tbsps maple syrup
- Mix all the ingredients together.

METHOD

Every day: Get your body moving gently; go for a walk or bike ride.

Day 1 and 2: Eat only raw or steamed fruit and vegetables on these two days. Drink at least two 7 fl oz/200 ml servings of "liver lemonade" and eight 7 fl oz/ 200 ml servings of water.

Day 3: Drink only water and fresh fruit juices on this day, along with at least four 7 fl oz/200 ml servings of "liver lemonade."

Day 4 = liver cleanse day: Drink at least four 7 fl oz/200 ml servings of "liver lemonade" and as much water as you like. Before going to bed, drink 1 tbsp cold-pressed organic olive oil followed by 7 fl oz/200 ml of "liver lemonade."

Day 5: Follow the same steps as for Day 3.

Day 6 and 7: Follow the same steps as for Days 1 and 2.

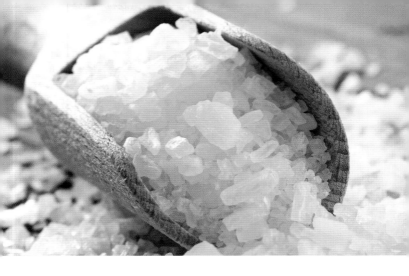

Sea salt bath

BACK-GROUND
Bathing is an ancient ritual with relaxing, calming, and health-giving effects on body and mind. Compared with other sea salts, salt from the Dead Sea is rich in magnesium and potassium but low in sodium chloride (cooking salt), and this is why salt from this source is so effective for therapeutic purposes.

EFFECT
A sea salt bath will calm the mind, ease rheumatic complaints, and soothe muscle cramps or stiffness. It can help with sciatica, joint pain, lumbago, and skin problems, while also boosting the circulation and relaxing the entire body.

METHOD

You will need 8 oz (250 g) of medicinal bath salts for a full bathtub of water. They are available from pharmacies, health food stores, or drugstores. Dissolve the salt in water that is as hot as possible, then top up with cold until the bathwater has reached an ideal temperature of about 100°F (38°C). Enjoy your bath for about 15 or 20 minutes After bathing, rinse your body with warm, unsalted water; don't use any soap. Take a quiet moment after your bath to rest for a while. One sea salt bath a week is enough to get the full benefit of the positive effects this will have for body and mind.

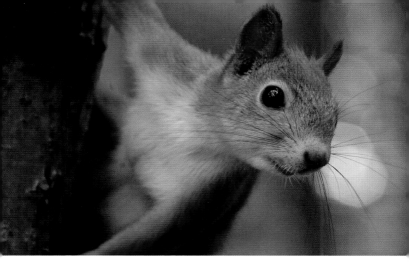

Energy nuts

BACK-GROUND
Nuts are an excellent source of energy and TCM teaches that walnuts in particular have highly beneficial effects on people's physical and mental health. Walnuts contain valuable proteins, carbohydrates, important minerals, and fiber, as well as higher concentrations of vitamins A, B, C, and E than are found in many varieties of fruit and vegetables.

EFFECT
As walnuts look very similar to the human brain, Chinese tradition maintains that eating them may have a positive effect on intelligence. Walnuts will also boost your primal energy and have beneficial effects on the kidneys, lungs, and heart. They strengthen your

81

skin and hair while also exerting a positive influence on the nerves and mind. Walnuts are nutritious, harmonizing, astringent, and anti-inflammatory, and they have the added advantage of reducing blood sugar levels.

Ingredients

- 2 cups (8 oz/200 g) peeled and halved walnuts
- 1 oz (20 g) sesame seeds
- 2–4 tbsps maple syrup

METHOD Dry fry the walnuts in a pan (without oil or butter), making sure the nuts do not burn. Pour the roasted walnuts into a dish, top them while still warm with maple syrup, and sprinkle the sesame seeds over the top. Mix everything up well and let the nuts cool. Store them in a container with a tight-fitting lid in a cool, dark place. Enjoy a handful of tasty energy nuts every day.

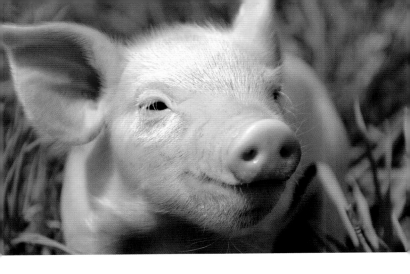

Nasal irrigation

BACKGROUND

Rinsing the nose with warm salt water is an old yogic exercise that is carried out every day for purification and hygiene reasons. It's like cleaning your teeth and has a preventive effect, but can also help soothe, for example, hay fever or a slight cold.

EFFECT

The warm salt water cleanses your nose, sinuses, and nasal mucosa. Rinsing your nose has a very positive effect on allergies such as hay fever or a house dust allergy. This simple technique boosts immune response, clears your airways, provides relief from a bunged-up or running nose, and is generally good for colds and inflammation of the sinus cavities.

METHOD

Rinse out your nose with warm salt water. You can buy little irrigators from specialist stores, and these will make it easier to pour water into your nose. To make the salt solution, mix a pinch (about 1 g) of salt into a scant half a cup (100 ml) of warm water. The salt should be properly dissolved in the water before you cleanse first one nostril and then the other with the saline solution. Clean up your nose with a tissue afterward. You can also buy ready-made cooking salt solutions for nasal irrigation in pharmacies and drugstores. Cleanse your nose daily; the best time is when you get up in the morning.

To take additional care of your nose, you can add one or two drops of oil to each nostril. Here, you can use either a pure oil, such as matured organic sesame oil, or a special herbal oil for the nose.

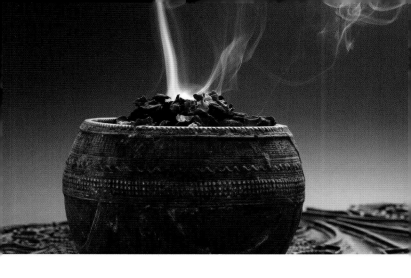

Cleansing your outer and inner worlds

Burning incense has been a common practice since ancient times, when it was performed mainly for religious purposes, as a sacrificial offering, or for disinfection purposes. Nowadays, it is principally used to purify the atmosphere, to aid concentration while meditating, to boost mental energy, and to work in conjunction with natural medicine.

EFFECT

Burning incense cancels negative vibrations, removes bad smells from your surroundings, and cleanses body and mind. It has the power to strengthen mood, and depending on the ingredients used, incense can purify, calm, heal, strengthen, stimulate, clarify, promote concentration, free the mind, and bring well-being. Burning incense stimulates the senses while centering and harmonizing both body and mind.

- *To cleanse the atmosphere,* suitable ingredients include frankincense, juniper, spruce, Scots pine, stone pine, lemon balm, clove, peppermint, eucalyptus, myrrh, camphor, and white sage.

- *For relaxing and harmonizing results,* suitable ingredients include cinnamon, sandalwood, agarwood, verbena, camomile, lavender, marjoram, cedar, and myrrh.

- *For energizing, strengthening, and invigorating results,* suitable ingredients include galangal, frankincense, mugwort, thyme, juniper, elecampane, angelica root, cardamom, lemon balm, and orange.

- *For cheering, antidepressant results,* suitable ingredients include cardamom, fennel, St John's wort, lemongrass, rose, patchouli, yerba santa, star anise, lemon balm, and cedarwood.

- *For meditative and spiritual results, or to promote concentration,* suitable ingredients include bay leaf, agarwood, rosemary, saffron, sandalwood, eucalyptus, clove, and frankincense.

METHOD Decide for yourself whether you prefer incense sticks or the traditional approach of burning incense over charcoal or in a little mesh basket. When buying incense, always take care that it contains no artificial additives or fillers, and has been manufactured from pure woods, resins, blossoms, and herbs. Create a small personal ritual, for example by selecting a scent that matches your needs or desires, and then burning incense in a room or the whole house. Try to maintain focus throughout the incense ritual, and accompany it with positive thoughts for even more enjoyable results. Air the room(s) just before and after burning incense.

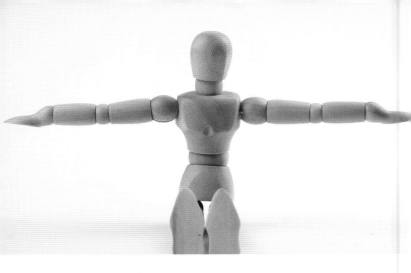

Rotating your joints

BACK-GROUND TCM holds that joints that are moved too little or in the wrong way can cause an increase in energy blocks and thereby exert a negative influence on the flow of qi throughout the body's entire energy system. A joint is like a node or a railroad switch. If energy begins to back up at the ankle, for example, the qi that is absorbed from the ground via the sole will only be able to flow into the upper and lower thigh at a reduced rate. This is why it is important for all the joints in the body to be mobilized, activated, and moved regularly, according to a plan.

EFFECT This simple exercise will loosen up and invigorate your whole body. It promotes energy flow and mobility, purges any deposited waste, and makes your body feel good all over.

METHOD This exercise should be carried out standing up. Each joint in turn is carefully, slowly, and consciously rotated five to ten times in each direction. Breathe in and out through your nose throughout the entire exercise, and keep a relaxed and natural smile on your lips.

1. Ankle
2. Knee
3. Hip
4. Shoulder
5. Elbow
6. Wrist
7. Finger joint
8. Neck (move your head forward and back, then to the left and right, and lay the head sideways before turning it gently).

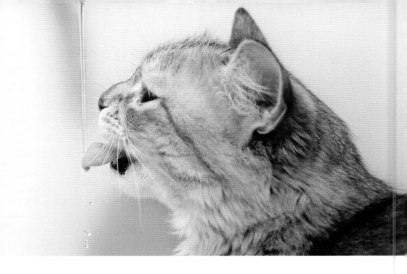

Cleansing your tongue

BACK-GROUND

The Ayurvedic tradition teaches that the tongue is closely linked to the gut through its organ reflex zones, and the toxins arising from a sluggish or poorly functioning metabolism will show up as a coating on the tongue.

EFFECT

This simple cleansing method will remove the mixture of toxins and bacteria that builds up on most people's tongues overnight and is deposited as a coating on its outer surface. This coating is often the cause of bad breath, caries, or periodontosis.

METHOD Take a little salt (cooking salt or sea salt) on your index finger and rub it all over your tongue before removing the coating with a small spoon or a tongue scraper, making sure you don't swallow the coating. Now clean your teeth or rinse your mouth with mouthwash.

To complement this technique, I recommend the exercises "Eye bath" (p. 9), "Oil pulling" (p. 29), and "Nasal irrigation" (p. 83).

Exercise routines

Here are my suggestions for a few exercise routines. The individual exercises build on one another in a structured way, each one helping with the next technique. I have selected and arranged the sequences in order to provide you with a self-contained and harmonized energy program that will make your vital physical and mental energy flow, but feel free to create your own programs by linking up the lists or combining different exercises. Keep a careful eye on how you are feeling, both physically and mentally, after each individual workout as well as at the end of the routine.

An energetic start to the day
- Oil pulling p. 29
- Cleansing your tongue
  p. 90
- Nasal irrigation p. 83
- Drinking hot water p. 19
- Rolling your feet p. 13
- Buddha's rice soup p. 49

Deep and restful sleep
- Primal scream p. 23
- A bath for the senses p. 66
- Cleansing your outer and
  inner worlds p. 85
- OM: A word of power p. 35

Strong nerves
- Alternate breathing p. 21
- Primal scream p. 23
- Tapping your thymus gland
  p. 11
- Nerve biscuits p. 58

A cheerful mood
- The power of a smile p. 43
- Bumble bee breath p. 68
- Walking backward p. 37
- A bath for the senses p. 66
- Cleansing your outer and
  inner worlds p. 85

Epilogue

Letting go is the art of freeing yourself physically, mentally, and materially of all unnecessary ballast. It lays the foundations for opening yourself up to life and to people, again and again. Life means constant flux and change, and only those who have learned to go with life's flow will be able to rid themselves of unnecessary pain and suffering. Clinging on to things, on the other hand, blocks the natural flow of energy, preventing development and progress. It is important to focus on the idea of letting go at regular intervals, so you can release new energy and reinvigorate sources of energy that have run dry. People who let go create space for new things, which can only come into your life when the old has been mastered. The more effectively you can let go on a physical and mental level, the more vital energy you will enjoy, the more you will be living from your inner core, and the more authentic you will be.

Energy knows no borders. It cannot be destroyed, it can only be transformed. The highest art in life is to use our energy correctly and with focus. Our energy flows when we give in, when we let go, when we give ourselves over to the flow of our lives. There are many ways and means that can help us here, and this little energy guide is one of them. I hope that the various exercises, techniques, and recipes will get the energy flowing in your mind and body, showing you the path that leads to yourself.

My very best wishes,
Sandy Taikyu Kuhn Shimu

Acknowledgment

Energy is omnipresent. It is revealed in trust and gratitude, and I would like to sincerely thank all those beings who have made it possible for this book to find its way to you. May the energy of this togetherness flow into our hearts and minds!

About the author

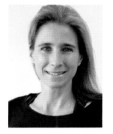

Sandy Taikyu Kuhn Shimu, Zen master, artist, and author, principally works as a teacher and educator in the fields of kung fu, yoga, qigong, and Zen, and as a counsellor. She has developed the WULIN principle and her own counselling methodology, WULIN Zen coaching. She is also a co-founder of the WULIN organization and of the WULIN approach to Zen. She is passionate about connecting with and applying traditional teachings in practical situations and the routines of modern life. Sandy Taikyu Kuhn Shimu finds fulfillment in her writing and her day-to-day tuition of pupils at home in Switzerland and abroad.

Further information about the author's activities is available from:

www.taikyu.ch
www.wulin.ch

Picture credits

Page 3: Igor Tarasov, 9: Thomas Francois, 11: Pabkov, 17: Barbara Helgason, 19: studiovespa, 23: k_tsygankova, 25: avs_lt, 27: xjrshimada, 29: Roman Thomas, 31: fotodesign-jegg.de, 35: ping han, 37: marylooo, 39: Michael Rekochinsky, 41: Helder Almeida, 43: Asray Laleike, 45: thingamajiggs, 49: airborne77, 52: pio3, 54: Javier brosch, 56: Svenja98, 58: unpict, 60: Argus, 62: NFSR, 64: HumerMedia, 66: gudrun, 68: Den, 70: sevenmultimedia, 72: Tanja, 74: yanlev, 79: HLPhoto, 81: mbongo, 85: LoSa, 88: FotoDesignPP, 90: Nataliya Dvukhimenna. All Adobe Stock (www.stock.adobe.com)

Page 13: Ilya.K, 15: Nathapol Kongseang, 21: coka, 33: Ekaterina Kondratova, 47: Billion Photos, 76: Maks Narodenko, 83: Volodymyr Burdiak. All shutterstock.com

For further information and to request a book catalog contact:
Inner Traditions, One Park Street, Rochester, Vermont 05767

Earthdancer Books is an Inner Traditions imprint.
Phone: +1-800-246-8648, customerservice@innertraditions.com
www.earthdancerbooks.com • www.innertraditions.com

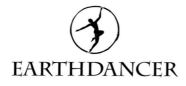

EARTHDANCER

AN INNER TRADITIONS IMPRINT